DIABETIC RENAL DIET COOKBOOK

FOR SENIORS

The Ultimate Guide with 20 Delicious & Easy Recipes for Managing Diabetes and Chronic Kidney Disease in Your Golden Years

Patricia Camire

CHECK OTHER BOOKS BY AUTHOR:

TABLE OF CONTENT

INTRODUCTION

Ms. Thompson, a lively senior facing the obstacles of diabetes and chronic kidney disease, began a change in her quiet kitchen with Patricia Camire's "Diabetic Renal Diet Cookbook for Seniors."

Faced with gastronomic uncertainty and the monotony of dietary limitations, Ms. Thompson discovered a world of sensations that did not jeopardize her health.

As she glanced through the cookbook, each page showed not just dishes but also a road map to health. The zesty lemon herb grilled chicken added a burst of freshness to her meal, while the avocado and black bean salsa offered a symphony of textures and nutrition.

Ms. Thompson expertly managed the culinary hurdles, transforming them into innovative possibilities.

The true magic happened when her biweekly check-ups revealed changes. Stable blood sugar levels and improved renal function became testaments to the cookbook's success.

For Ms. Thompson, the cookbook was more than simply a compilation of recipes; it was a guide on her path to wellness, demonstrating that every delicious mouthful might be a step toward a better and more vibrant existence.

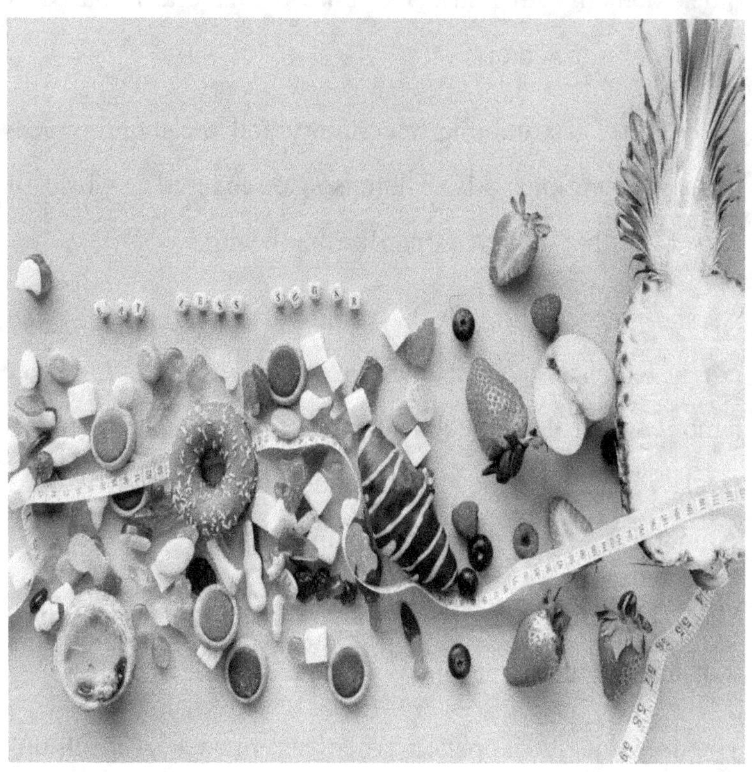

CHAPTER ONE

GENERAL OVERVIEW OF DIABETIC RENAL DIET

Understanding Diabetic Renal Health

Diabetes and chronic kidney disease (CKD) are two interrelated health issues that frequently coexist, especially in the elderly population. This Chapter of the "Diabetic Renal Diet Cookbook for Seniors" provides as a starting point, diving into the complexities of these illnesses and highlighting the critical role nutrition plays in their management.

Introduction to Diabetic Renal Health

The trip begins with an investigation of the complex interaction between diabetes and chronic renal disease. Diabetes, which is defined by high blood sugar levels, can have a long-term impact on kidney function.

Chronic renal disease, on the other hand, is the steady loss of kidney function, which can be aggravated by uncontrolled diabetes.

The chapter begins with a poignant question: How can seniors handle the junction of these two health problems while yet embracing a healthy lifestyle?

The introduction establishes the tone for the entire chapter, emphasizing the need of following a diabetic renal diet, particularly in the golden years.

It is a call to action for seniors, urging them to take an active role in their health by making educated food decisions.

Diabetic Renal Diet Essentials

Navigating the complexities of a diabetic renal diet necessitates an awareness of the critical nutrients required for general health. This section delves into these elements, offering light on the delicate balance needed to properly treat diabetes and chronic renal disease.

This investigation will be built on guidelines for treating diabetes and CKD through food choices. It is not simply limiting particular foods, but rather adopting a comprehensive approach to nutrition.

The talk includes the effects of sodium, potassium, and phosphorus on renal function, giving seniors vital insights for adjusting their diets to individual health needs.

This part becomes a practical guide for seniors, providing them with the information they need to make educated decisions about their daily food habits.

It establishes the foundation for a tailored approach to nutrition, emphasizing that each plate represents a chance to contribute to better health.

Culinary Challenges and Solutions for Seniors

Transitioning to a specialized diet can be difficult, especially for seniors. In this part, the chapter confronts these culinary challenges head on.

It recognizes the reality of aging—possible movement limits, changes in taste perception, and the necessity for reduced meal preparation.

Practical suggestions for meal planning, grocery shopping, and cooking are featured prominently. These ideas are both educational and sensitive, acknowledging the specific conditions that elders may confront.

The idea is to turn significant roadblocks into doable chores, making adopting a diabetic renal diet a viable and fun activity.

Furthermore, unique solutions are interwoven into the story. Cooking becomes an art form, and seniors are encouraged to try new flavors, experiment with herbs and spices, and enjoy the culinary experience.

The part attempts to boost seniors' confidence by encouraging them to see their kitchen as a place for food and self-expression.

Benefits of Diabetic Renal Diet for Seniors

As the chapter progresses, the focus changes to the benefits that a well-balanced diabetic renal diet may provide. It is not just about treating illnesses, but also about improving general health and well-being.

The advantages of following a diabetic renal diet go beyond the avoidance of problems. The tale includes real-life success stories—testimonials from seniors who have flourished on such diets, reporting higher energy, lower blood sugar levels, and better renal function.

These experiences serve as beacons of hope, demonstrating that a diabetic renal diet is not a limiting measure, but rather a road to a more robust and meaningful existence.

Seniors are urged to see their food choices as a way of recovering control over their health. Adopting a diabetic renal diet is a path of empowerment, allowing patients to actively engage in their own health.

The positivism incorporated into this part acts as a motivator, encouraging seniors to embrace the potential for good change via their food choices.

In essence, this chapter serves as the foundation for the rest of the book. It's a complete handbook that both informs and inspires.

It pave the way for seniors to go on a culinary experience that goes beyond the confines of health management, allowing them to appreciate the richness of life via tasty, nutritious, and purposeful meals.

The story unfolds with compassion, acknowledging seniors' specific problems and successes while also providing a road map for navigating the complex landscape of diabetic renal health.

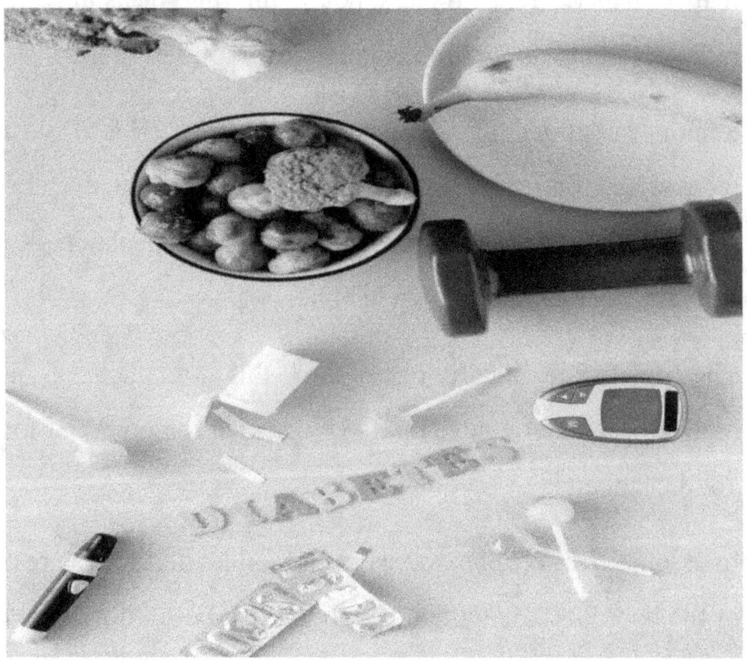

CHAPTER TWO

DELICIOUS DIABETIC RENAL DIET RECIPES

1. Herb-Roasted Salmon with Lemon Quinoa

Ingredients:

- 4 salmon fillets

- 1 tablespoon olive oil

- 1 teaspoon dried thyme

- 1 teaspoon of dry rosemary

- 1 teaspoon dried parsley

- Add salt and pepper to taste

- Rinse 1 cup of quinoa,

- Zest and juice of 1 lemon

- 2 cups of low-sodium chicken broth

- Chopped fresh parsley for garnish

Instructions:

1. Preheat your oven to 375°F (190°C).

2. Arrange the salmon fillets on a baking pan lined with parchment paper.

3. In a small bowl, combine the olive oil, dried thyme, dry rosemary, dried parsley, salt, and pepper.

4. Brush the herb mixture on the fish fillets.

5. Bake for 15-20 minutes, or until the salmon is well cooked and readily flaked.

6. In a saucepan, mix the quinoa, lemon zest, lemon juice, and chicken broth.

7. Bring to a boil, then decrease heat, cover, and simmer for 15-20 minutes, or until the quinoa is done.

8. Serve the herb-roasted fish with lemon quinoa and fresh parsley.

2. Cabbage and Carrot Stir-Fry with Tofu

Ingredients:

- Thinly sliced 1 small cabbage,

- Julienned 2 carrots,

- 1 block cubed of extra-firm tofu,

- 2 tablespoons of low-sodium soy sauce

- 1 tablespoon of sesame oil

- 1 teaspoon of minced ginger

- 2 chopped garlic cloves

- 1 tablespoon of rice vinegar

- 1 tablespoon chopped green onions for garnish

Instructions:

1. Heat sesame oil in a wok or pan over medium heat.

2. Sauté the minced ginger and garlic for 1-2 minutes, until aromatic.

3. Cook the tofu cubes until golden brown on all sides.

4. Stir in the chopped cabbage and julienned carrots, simmering until tender-crisp.

5. In a small dish, combine the soy sauce and rice vinegar, then add to the stir-fry.

6. Toss everything together until evenly coated and cooked through.

7. Just before serving, garnish with chopped green onion.

3. Berry and Almond Chia Pudding

Ingredients:

- 1/4 cup chia seeds

- 1 cup of unsweetened almond milk

- 1/2 teaspoon of vanilla extract

- 1 tablespoon of almond butter

- 1 cup of mixed berries such as strawberries, blueberries, or raspberries

- 1 tablespoon of chopped almonds

Instructions:

1. In a dish, combine chia seeds, almond milk, vanilla essence, and almond butter.

2. Allow it to settle for 15-20 minutes, stirring regularly, until it has thickened into a pudding-like consistency.

3. Place the chia pudding in serving cups and top with mixed berries.

4. Repeat the layers, finishing with chopped almonds.

5. Store at a low temperature for minimum of 2 hours or overnight.

6. Serve chilled and enjoy this delicious and kidney-friendly dessert.

4. Spinach and Mushroom Quiche with Sweet Potato Crust

Ingredients:

- 2 medium sweet potatoes, peeled and thinly sliced

- Cut 1 cup of fresh spinach

- Slice 1 cup of mushrooms,

- 4 big eggs

- One cup of unsweetened almond milk

- Season with Salt and pepper to make it sweet

- Add 1/2 teaspoon of garlic powder

- 1/2 teaspoon of onion powder

- 1/4 cup shredded Parmesan cheese (optional)

Instructions:

1. Preheat your oven to 375°F (190°C).

2. Arrange sweet potato slices in a pie plate to make a crust.

3. In a pan, cook the mushrooms and spinach until softened.

4. In a bowl, combine the eggs, almond milk, salt, pepper, garlic powder, and onion powder.

5. Spread the sautéed veggies over the sweet potato crust.

6. Empty the egg mixture on the veggies.

7. Optional: sprinkle Parmesan cheese over top.

8. Bake for 30–35 minutes, or until the quiche is set and golden brown.

5. Lemon Herb Grilled Chicken with Cauliflower Rice

Ingredients:

- 4 boneless and skinless chicken breasts

- Zest and juice from two lemons

- 2 tablespoons of olive oil

- 1 teaspoon of dried oregano

- 1 teaspoon of dried thyme

- 1 teaspoon of paprika

- Season with Salt and pepper to make it sweet

- Grate one head of cauliflower to resemble rice.

- 2 tablespoons of chopped fresh parsley for garnish

Instructions:

1. In a bowl, combine the lemon zest, lemon juice, olive oil, oregano, thyme, paprika, salt, and pepper.

2. Marinate the chicken breasts in the marinade for 30 minutes.

3. Grill the chicken until thoroughly done, about 6-8 minutes per side.

4. While the chicken is frying, cook the grated cauliflower in a skillet until soft.

5. Serve the grilled chicken over cauliflower rice.

6. Before serving, garnish with finely chopped parsley.

6. Broccoli and Walnut Salad with Balsamic Vinaigrette

Ingredients:

- 2 cups of blanched broccoli florets,

- 1/2 cup of chopped walnuts,

- 1/4 cup of finely chopped red onion,

- 1/4 cup crumbled feta cheese (optional)

- To make the dressing, combine 2 tablespoons balsamic vinegar

- 1 tablespoon of olive oil

- 1 teaspoon of Dijon mustard

- Salt and pepper to taste

Instructions:

1. In a bowl, add blanched broccoli, walnuts, red onion, and feta cheese.

2. In a small jar, combine the balsamic vinegar, olive oil, Dijon mustard, salt, and pepper to make the vinaigrette.

3. Toss the salad with the vinaigrette until well coated.

4. Allow the flavors to blend for at least 15 minutes before serving.

7. Turkey and Vegetable Skewers with Cilantro-Lime Quinoa

Ingredients:

- 1 pound turkey breast (cut into bits)

- Slice one zucchini and chop one bell pepper into bits

- One red onion, sliced into wedges

- Two tablespoons of olive oil

- Add 1 teaspoon ground cumin

- 1 teaspoon smoked paprika

- Add Salt and pepper to taste

- Cook 1 cup of quinoa

- Zest and juice One lime

- Fresh cilantro as garnish

Instructions:

1. Preheat your grill or grill pan.

2. In a mixing dish, combine turkey pieces, zucchini, bell pepper, and red onion with olive oil, cumin, smoked paprika, salt, and pepper.

3. Thread the seasoned turkey and veggies on skewers.

4. Grill the skewers for 8-10 minutes, rotating regularly, until the turkey is well cooked.

5. In a separate dish, combine cooked quinoa, lime zest, and juice.

6. Top the turkey and veggie skewers with cilantro-lime quinoa and sprinkle with fresh cilantro.

8. Cauliflower and Broccoli Soup with Herbed Greek Yogurt

Ingredients:

- 1 chopped head cauliflower,

- 2 cups of broccoli florets

- Dice one onion

- Mince two cloves garlic

- 4 cups of low-sodium vegetable broth

- 1 teaspoon of dried thyme

- 1 teaspoon of dried oregano

- Season with Salt and pepper to add flavour

- Add 1/2 cup of plain Greek yogurt

- Fresh chives as garnish

Instructions:

1. In a large saucepan, cook the chopped onion and minced garlic until tender.

2. Add the chopped cauliflower, broccoli florets, vegetable broth, thyme, oregano, salt, and pepper to the saucepan.

3. Bring to a boil, then decrease the heat and simmer until the veggies are cooked.

4. Using an immersion blender, mix the soup until smooth.

5. In a small dish, combine Greek yogurt and dry herbs.

6. Serve the soup hot, garnished with herbed Greek yogurt and fresh chives.

9. Grilled Eggplant and Tomato Salad with Basil Vinaigrette

Ingredients:

- 2 medium sliced eggplants,

- 2 cups of halved cherry tomatoes,

- 1/4 cup balsamic vinegar

- 1/4 cup olive oil

- 1 tablespoon of Dijon mustard

- 1 teaspoon honey, salt, and pepper to taste

- Garnish with fresh basil leaves

Instructions:

1. Preheat your grill or grill pan.

2. Brush eggplant slices with olive oil and grill until cooked, 3-4 minutes per side.

3. Whisk together balsamic vinegar, olive oil, Dijon mustard, honey, salt, and pepper to make the vinaigrette.

4. Place the grilled eggplant pieces and cherry tomatoes in a serving plate.

5. Drizzle the salad with the basil vinaigrette and mix gently.

6. Just before serving, garnish with fresh basil leaves.

10. Lemon Garlic Shrimp Stir-Fry with Asparagus

Ingredients:

- 1 pound of skinned and deveined shrimp

- 1 bunch of trimmed and chopped asparagus into bite-sized pieces

- Two teaspoons of olive oil

- 3 garlic cloves, minced

- Zest and juice from 1 lemon

- One teaspoon of low-sodium soy sauce

- One teaspoon honey

- Add Salt and pepper to taste

- Serve with brown rice or cauliflower rice

Instructions:

1. Warm olive oil in a wok or pan over medium-high heat.

2. Add the minced garlic and simmer until fragrant.

3. Add the shrimp and asparagus to the pan, stirring constantly until the shrimp turn pink and opaque.

4. In a small bowl, combine the lemon zest, lemon juice, soy sauce, honey, salt, and pepper.

5. Toss the shrimp and asparagus with the sauce until well coated.

6. Serve the lemon garlic shrimp stir-fry with brown or cauliflower rice.

11. Quinoa Salad with Chickpeas and Roasted Vegetables

Ingredients:

- 1 cup of cooked quinoa,

- 1 can (15 oz) of drained and rinsed chickpeas,

- 1 diced zucchini,

- 1 diced red bell pepper,

- 1 cup of halved cherry tomatoes,

- 2 tablespoons of olive oil

- 1 teaspoon of dried basil

- 1 teaspoon of dried oregano

- Add Salt and pepper to taste

- Feta cheese (optional) as garnish

Instructions:

1. Preheat your oven to 400°F (200°C).

2. In a mixing dish, combine chopped zucchini, red bell pepper, and cherry tomatoes with olive oil, dried basil, dry oregano, salt, and pepper.

3. Place the veggies on a baking pan and roast for 20-25 minutes, until brown.

4. In a large bowl, mix the cooked quinoa, chickpeas, and roasted veggies.

5. Drizzle with more olive oil if preferred and toss to blend.

6. Just before serving, garnish with crumbled feta cheese.

12. Baked Cod with Herbed Tomato Salsa

Ingredients:

- 4 cod fillets

- 2 cups of cherry tomatoes, quartered

- 1/4 cup of chopped fresh basil,

- 1/4 cup of chopped fresh parsley,

- 1 tablespoon of olive oil

- 1 tablespoon of balsamic vinegar

- 2 minced garlic cloves

- Salt and pepper to taste

- Lemon wedges to serve

Instructions:

1. Preheat oven to 400°F (200°C).

2. Arrange the fish fillets on a baking pan lined with parchment paper.

3. In a mixing bowl, add the quartered cherry tomatoes, basil, parsley, olive oil, balsamic vinegar, minced garlic, salt, and pepper.

4. Spoon the herbed tomato salsa over the fish fillets.

5. Bake the fish for 15-20 minutes, or until well done.

6. Serve the cooked fish with herbed tomato salsa and lemon wedges.

13. Lentil and Vegetable Stew

Ingredients:

- 1 cup dried green lentils, washed

- 4 cups of low-sodium vegetable broth

- 1 chopped onion

- 2 diced carrots,

- 2 diced celery stalks,

- 2 minced garlic cloves

- Add 1 teaspoon of ground cumin

- 1 teaspoon of smoked paprika

- Add Salt and pepper to taste

- Garnish with fresh parsley

Instructions:

1. In a large saucepan, add lentils, vegetable broth, onion, carrots, celery, garlic, cumin, smoked paprika, salt, and pepper.

2. Bring to a boil, then decrease the heat and simmer for 25-30 minutes, or until the lentils and veggies are cooked.

3. Adjust the seasoning as needed.

4. Sprinkle with fresh parsley before serving.

14. Grilled Chicken and Vegetable Kebabs with Lemon Herb Marinade

Ingredients:

- 1 pound boneless, skinless chicken breasts (cut into bits).

- 1 zucchini, cut

- 1 yellow bell pepper, sliced into bits

- 1 red onion, sliced into wedges

- Two teaspoons of olive oil

- Zest and juice from 1 lemon

- Use 1 teaspoon of dried thyme

- 1 teaspoon of dry rosemary

- Add Salt and pepper to taste

Instructions:

1. Preheat grill or grill pan.

2. In a bowl, combine the olive oil, lemon zest, lemon juice, dried thyme, dried rosemary, salt, and pepper.

3. Thread chicken chunks, zucchini slices, bell pepper chunks, and red onion wedges on skewers.

4. Brush the kebabs with the lemon herb marinade.

5. Grill for 8-10 minutes, turning regularly, until the chicken is fully cooked and the veggies are soft.

15. Roasted Butternut Squash and Quinoa Salad

Ingredients:

- 2 cups chopped butternut

- 1 cup of cooked quinoa,

- 1/4 cup of dried cranberries

- 1/4 cup of chopped pecans

- 2 tablespoons of olive oil

- 1 tablespoon of balsamic vinegar

- 1 teaspoon of maple syrup

- Add Salt and pepper to taste

- Garnish with fresh kale leaves

Instructions:

1. Preheat your oven to 400°F (200°C).

2. Toss diced butternut squash with olive oil, salt, and pepper, then roast for 20-25 minutes, or until golden and soft.

3. In a mixing dish, add cooked quinoa, roasted butternut squash, dried cranberries, and chopped pecans.

4. In a small jar, combine olive oil, balsamic vinegar, maple syrup, salt, and pepper to make the dressing.

5. Drizzle the salad with the dressing and toss to mix.

6. Just before serving, garnish with fresh kale leaves.

16. Asian-Inspired Salmon and Vegetable Stir-Fry

Ingredients:

- 4 salmon fillets

- 2 cups of broccoli florets

- 1 sliced red bell pepper,

- 1 cup of snap peas, trimmed

- Two tablespoons low-sodium soy sauce

- 1 tablespoon of hoisin sauce

- 1 tablespoon of sesame oil

- 1 teaspoon of grated ginger

- 2 chopped garlic cloves

- One tablespoon of olive oil

- Sesame seeds as garnish

Instructions:

1. In a bowl, combine soy sauce, hoisin sauce, sesame oil, grated ginger, and chopped garlic.

2. Cut fish into bits and marinate in sauce for 15-20 minutes.

3. In a wok or pan, heat olive oil over medium-high heat.

4. Place the marinated salmon, broccoli, red bell pepper, and snap peas in the pan.

5. Stir-fry until the salmon is cooked through and the veggies are soft and crispy.

6. Just before serving, garnish with sesame seeds.

17. Quinoa and Black Bean Stuffed Peppers

Ingredients:

- 4 halved bell peppers with seeds removed

- 1 cup of cooked quinoa,

- 1 can (15 oz) drained and rinsed black beans

- 1 cup of corn kernels

- 1 cup of cherry tomatoes, diced

- 1 teaspoon of ground cumin

- 1 teaspoon of chili powder

- Add Salt and pepper to taste

- Garnish with fresh cilantro

Instructions:

1. Preheat your oven to 375°F (190°C).

2. In a bowl, add the cooked quinoa, black beans, corn, cherry tomatoes, ground cumin, chili powder, salt, and pepper.

3. Fill each bell pepper half with quinoa mixture.

4. Arrange the filled peppers in a baking dish and cover with aluminum foil.

5. Cook in the oven for 25–30 minutes, or until the peppers are tender.

6. Before serving, garnish with chopped fresh cilantro.

18. Turkey and Vegetable Curry with Cauliflower Rice

Ingredients:

- 1 pound meat turkey

- 1 cauliflower, shredded to resemble rice

- 1 finely chopped onion,

- 2 diced carrots,

- 1 cup of chopped green beans,

- 1 can (14 oz) of coconut milk

- 2 tablespoons of red curry paste

- 1 tablespoon of olive oil

- 1 teaspoon of turmeric

- Add Salt and pepper to taste

- Garnish with fresh cilantro

Instructions:

1. In a large pan, increase the olive oil temperature over medium heat.

2. Add the chopped onion and heat until softened.

3. Add the ground turkey and heat until browned.

4. Add diced carrots and cut green beans.

5. In a small bowl, combine the coconut milk, red curry paste, turmeric, salt, and pepper.

6. Pour the curry sauce over the turkey and veggies, then cook until the vegetables are soft.

7. In a separate skillet, cook the grated cauliflower until it resembles rice.

8. Serve the turkey and vegetable curry over cauliflower rice, topped with fresh cilantro.

19. Eggplant and Tomato Casserole with Herbed Quinoa

Ingredients:

- 1 sliced large eggplant,

- 2 cups of halved cherry tomatoes,

- 1 cup of cooked quinoa,

- 1/4 cup of chopped fresh basil

- 2 tablespoons of olive oil

- 1 teaspoon of dried oregano

- Add Salt and pepper to taste

- 1/4 cup grated Parmesan cheese (optional)

Instructions:

1. Preheat oven to 375°F (190°C).

2. Arrange the eggplant slices in a baking tray.

3. In a mixing dish, combine cherry tomatoes, cooked quinoa, chopped basil, olive oil, dried oregano, salt, and pepper.

4. Spread the quinoa-tomato mixture over the eggplant pieces.

5. If desired, add grated Parmesan cheese on top.

6. Bake for 25-30 minutes, or until the eggplant is soft and the top is golden brown.

20. Mediterranean Chickpea Salad with Lemon Vinaigrette

Ingredients:

- Two cans of chickpeas (15 oz each), drained and rinsed

- 1 cucumber, diced

- 1 cup of halved cherry tomatoes,

- 1/2 finely chopped red onion,

- 1/4 cup of sliced Kalamata olives,

- Use 1/4 cup of crumbled feta cheese

- 2 tablespoons olive oil

- Zest and juice from 1 lemon

- One teaspoon of dried oregano

- Add Salt and pepper to taste

- Garnish with fresh parsley

Instructions:

1. In a large mixing bowl, add chickpeas, diced cucumber, split cherry tomatoes, chopped red onion, sliced Kalamata olives, and crumbled feta cheese.

2. In a small jar, combine olive oil, lemon zest, lemon juice, dried oregano, salt, and pepper to make the vinaigrette.

3. Toss the chickpea salad with the lemon vinaigrette until coated.

4. Sprinkle with fresh parsley before serving.

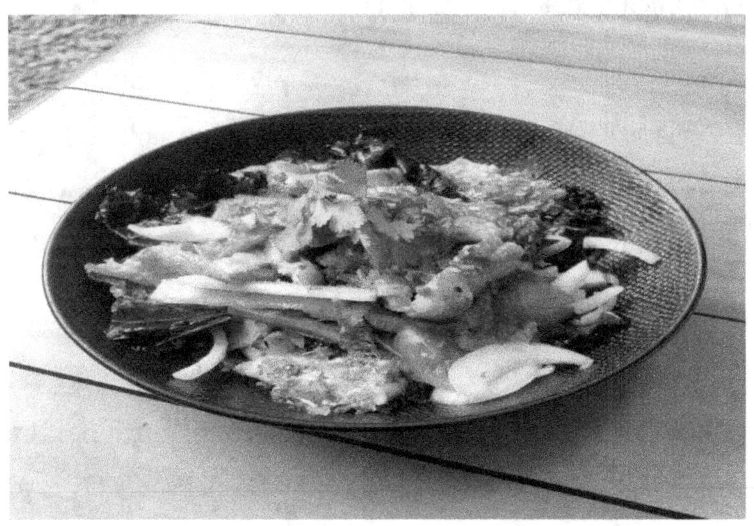

CONCLUSION

We conclude our Diabetic Renal Diet Cookbook for Seniors by celebrating the wonderful mix of healthy options and delightful flavors.

Each formula is meticulously created, taking into account the specific requirements of diabetes management and kidney health.

As we traveled across different culinary environments, the emphasis on kidney-friendly foods, balanced nutrition, and enjoyment remained consistent.

This cookbook is more than simply a compilation of recipes; it's a guide to living a healthy and meaningful life. It enables seniors to enjoy the richness of life while prioritizing their health by providing healthful, mindfully crafted meals.

May each meal be a testament to the joy that comes from nourishing both body and spirit, demonstrating that healthy eating can be a pleasant and rewarding endeavor. Cheers to a delicious, nutritious, and heart-healthy trip ahead!

Thank you for starting your culinary journey with the Diabetic Renal Diet Cookbook for Seniors. Your dedication to putting health first and enjoying excellent meals encourages us.

This cookbook is more than just a compilation of recipes; it's a passionate guide for improving your health and bringing joy into your kitchen.

We appreciate your faith in our ability to create healthy and delectable solutions that address both diabetes control and renal health.

May these recipes give you energy, satisfaction, and a fresh awareness for the link between good food and a healthy lifestyle. Here's to your well-being, happiness, and many more wonderful times ahead.

With gratitude,

Patricia Camire

HAPPY COOKING!